YOUR BODY, A USER'S MANUAL

Your Body

A User's Manual

**How Real Men Work
without Pain, Booze,
or Drugs**

Dr. Laurie Meinholz

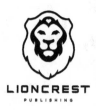

LIONCREST
PUBLISHING

YOUR BODY, A USER'S MANUAL

How Real Men Work without Pain, Booze, or Drugs

ISBN 978-1-5445-1919-7 *Paperback*
      978-1-5445-1918-0 *Ebook*

To all those who have self-medicated
and worked through the pain.

Contents

Introduction

Ben was repairing a piece of machinery on the farm and felt his lower back pop. He was unable to stand up straight and had severe muscle spasms, and he became frustrated because he had done similar repairs before and never had this severe an issue. In the past, when Ben had lower back pain, he was always able to work through it, and eventually it would stop hurting. But this time, it was not improving no matter what he did.

He picked up his tools, put everything away the best he could, and then returned home. When he arrived home, his wife Sara immediately knew that he needed to go to the chiropractor. Since Sara was a regular patient of mine, she knew he had to get help right away. She called my cell phone after hours. I told them I would meet them at my office, Nordic Chiropractic, as soon as they could get there. Although they lived only about fifteen minutes from downtown, it would take Ben about an hour to get in the car and get to my office. Since Ben was unable to sit down without severe pain, Sara took out the minivan's back seats. Ben stayed bent forward, crawled into the back of the van through the rear hatch, and lay down.

I was waiting at the office for them. When I saw them pull up, Sara opened the back hatch of the van and asked about the best way to get him into the office. I responded, "The same way he got into the van."

Ben looked hesitantly at me and said, "This is going to take me a while."

"That's okay," I said. "I don't have any plans for today."

Ben slowly inched out of the van and walked into my office, bent at the waist, looking straight down at the floor. The crown of his head leading him into the room, he couldn't stand straight enough to look me in the eyes. His speech was short and harsh; he answered my questions as directly as possible. He told me multiple times, "I don't care what you do; just fix me!" Muscle spasms took him fully to the ground in pain halfway through the visit, and I helped him return to a standing position. For parts of the visit, I lay on the floor next to him because he was too weak to sit or stand.

After the adjustment, Ben was able to stand upright, slowly walk out of the office, and sit in the van's passenger seat for the ride home. He was still in pain, but already his mobility was much improved. The next day, he came in for three different appointments. Rarely do I work on someone three times in the same day, but in severe cases, it can be necessary. With each visit, he improved significantly, and two days after the initial injury, he returned to full-time farm work, pain free.

After Ben got fixed up, he started to come in once a month to prevent this from happening again. When I met him, I didn't know he was addicted to drugs and alcohol, attending AA, and had been arrested occasionally for a DUI. To me, he was a typical farmer who threw out his lower back. About a year later, Ben visited me and told me that he was getting his six-month chip with AA that night. I congratulated him, and then he mumbled, "Thanks."

I thought I did not hear him correctly, so I said, "I'm sorry, what did you just say?"

He said, "I said, 'Thanks.'"

I told him, "Don't thank me! You're the one who has been sober for six months!"

Ben explained: Prior to coming in for his first adjustment, his back pain was so intense that he would often drink through his workday in order to dull the pain. He also explained that it was very isolating. Oftentimes, he would be stuck at home while his family or friends went out, so he would drink away the loneliness. Now that his back was not constantly hurting, he didn't have to self-medicate with alcohol.

This conversation happened three years ago. Ben

is still sober to this day. He comes in regularly—especially when he wants to drink, do drugs, or is in pain from working.

What I love about Ben's story is that it shows that when you are able to live pain free, every other aspect of your life automatically improves.

Ben admits, now that he is pain-free and sober, that he is a better farmer, able to work the overtime needed to finish the jobs, and a better husband and father.

I bet almost everyone reading this right now can think of someone like Ben. Maybe the person in your mind always has a doctor's appointment scheduled. They're always trying to figure out what is wrong, yet they never get any answers. Maybe they are always getting hurt on the job. If that person cannot do their job properly, they are suffering at home as well. Are they able to spend quality time with their kids? Spouse? Friends? Probably not. Are they able to help their spouse with work around the house? Are they able to sit on the bleachers through their kids' sporting events?

Living a pain-free life does not just impact the person who is in pain. It impacts their family, co-workers, and everyone else they interact with. When we are pain free, we are less likely to turn to drugs or alcohol. When we are pain free, we improve at work and with our families. It is when we are able to enjoy time with our family and friends and contribute at work that the whole community improves.

BECOMING A MECHANIC

I come from a family mainly made up of construction workers, landscapers, tradespeople, and dairy farmers. My dad was an ironworker/welder by trade. Growing up, I watched him having to work long hours during shutdowns, overtime, and holidays to pay the bills. I also grew up watching my dad get hurt on the job, from minor injuries to falling and breaking his back. As a result, he took many trips to the chiropractor over the years to keep himself working and living pain free. Many of his co-workers were in constant pain and/or addicted to drugs and alcohol. This is when I initially learned that the body's best mechanic is a chiropractor.

Although I grew up with my dad making regular trips to the chiropractor, I never pictured myself being a chiropractor. I attended Luther College, and after graduation, I ended up working as a receptionist in a chiropractic office in Waunakee, Wisconsin. I noticed that when people walked in, they were hurting and irritable. I could see the hurt in their eyes. After their adjustment from the chiropractor, I could see their relief. I could see them come alive again from the inside out.

Two weeks into working there, I knew I would become a chiropractor. I had no idea what was required for schooling, how much it would cost, where I would have to attend, or even if I could get into chiropractic college, but I knew that I had to become a chiropractor.

Even though I had seen many adjustments on my dad and other family members, I started asking the chiropractors I worked with questions like, "What do you *really* do in there?", "How does that help though?" and "How do you know what to do?" On slow days, I volunteered to write notes for the chiropractor during adjustments, so I could watch what they were really doing.

One year after I started working in the chiropractic office, I started classes at Palmer College of Chiropractic in Davenport, Iowa.

Now, as a chiropractor, I view myself as a mechanic for the body. I love helping people like Ben and like my dad get out of pain. I am so grateful to know how to improve our community by helping people get out of pain. I hope that this book will help you stop compromising your life and start living pain free.

CHAPTER 1

Your "Check Engine" Light Is On!

Imagine having to go to work as a construction worker and trying to get your job done while you have a pounding headache. All that you hear inside your head all day is thud, thud, thud. The whole time your head is pounding, your co-workers are pounding nails and running power tools right next to you, hollering to each other on the job site. Throughout the day, you load up on painkillers to ease the pain, but there is no change in your headache. You go home at night and try to play with your kids, be a good husband, and do yard work, but your headache is still there. You go to bed, finally fall asleep, and wake up again the next morning with the same headache. It is there all day at work and follows you home again. It is there when you try to play with your kids. It is there when you go to bed at night and wake up in the morning.

This goes on for twenty-five years.

Through the years, you try different over-the-counter medications, but none of them help. You try prescription drugs, but they do not lessen the pain. Then you try acupuncture, massage therapy, physical therapy, and targeting pressure points. Nothing helps. After a few years, you get concerned and go for an MRI just to be sure you don't have a tumor, but everything looks fine. While you are relieved that the MRI is clear, you are still haunted by the headache. At this point, all you're looking for is an answer, no matter how bad the news may be.

Having a daily pounding headache is your new normal. You know that nobody can help. You tell yourself that you are just unlucky. It must be your genetics. You must be getting old. Through the years, you consider switching professions, but this is the only skill you know.

Then, somehow, you end up at a chiropractor. You don't think it will help, but you figure it cannot hurt anything. After your first spinal adjustment, the twenty-five-year-old headache loosens its grip on you before you even get home.

You haven't had a headache since.

I know that there are many people out there who struggle with constant headaches. In fact, 85 percent of headaches are caused by spinal stress that can be improved with a single adjustment.

I do not like to see people suffer. Seeing people suffer is one of the hardest parts of my job. But I do like it when people are in pain. Yes, you read that right. I like it when people are in pain. Pain is a good thing to feel. Pain alerts us that something is going wrong within the body. From there, you have to find out *why* you have the pain, so it does not turn into chronic pain.

There are two rules in my office. When you are hurt or sick:

1. You cannot blame being old.
2. You cannot blame genetics.

Every day in the United States, we are told that the older we get, the more aches and pains we should have. This statement is both true and false. If you take care of your body when you are young, you should not hurt as you age. If you do not take care of your body and allow problems to pile up, then yes, the older you get, the more of a problem they become and the more pain you will have. Pain is not related to the aging process but to how well you have maintained your body over the years. With proper maintenance, you can live pain free. Even if you have not taken care of your body, it's never too late to start.

Believe it or not, your body is actually designed to become healthier and stronger as you age. Not weaker.

There are cultures in the world where the strongest and most fit people are the elders. One example is the Tarahumara tribe in Mexico. In this tribe, those who are over fifty are faster and stronger runners. The older people will run with, train, and teach the younger runners.[1] Contrast this to the US culture, where we mostly believe that, at fifty, you are considered old and incapable when it comes to physical strength. In the US, we tell people at fifty, "Slow down and don't use your body so much!"—whereas the Tarahumara tribe says the exact opposite. It is because of cultures like this that I do not allow patients to blame pain on their age.

There are very few genetic conditions that can cause pain and sickness. The majority of people do not have them. We will get more into this later.

Here is one thing I want you to understand: you have pain for a reason. Every single thing the body does, it does for a reason. Remember, your body never does anything by accident and never does anything wrong.

Pain is easy to brush off. You could say that pain is the body's way of punishing you or that your

---

1   Christopher McDougall, *Born to Run* (New York: Vintage Books, 2009).

body does not like you. But the body does not give you pain to spite you or make you miserable. Your body does not put you through more pain simply because you are aging. You do not get pain due to bad luck or because your parents had the same pain. And for the majority of people, you do not inherit pain from your bad genetics. There are a few genetic conditions that can cause an increased amount of pain, but so few of these exist that I do not allow anyone to blame their pain on their genetics.

When people feel pain, their instinct is to get rid of the pain as soon as possible. The worse the pain is, the more desperate they are to get rid of it. When people are in this state of mind, they don't care what rids them of the pain, as long as it goes away, even if relief is only temporary. It could be pain pills, massages, herbs, medical marijuana, muscle relaxers, *Biofreeze*, alcohol, illegal drugs, prescription drugs, etc. Oftentimes the body just flushes these out of the system, so the cycle continues.

While getting out of pain is always the goal, we need to make sure we don't get out of pain too soon. Pain is one of the ways that our body communicates with us. Pain is also how the body limits us from making the injury worse.

Throwing out your lower back is a great example. I know, from personal experience, it hurts a *lot*. When I threw out my lower back, my muscle spasms were so bad that I could not stand up straight and had to crawl into my chiropractor's office. Although painful, those muscle spasms were a protective mechanism to make sure the injury did not get worse or create any more damage; therefore, taking muscle relaxers is not the best idea because it allows more movement leading to further injury. If you add pain medication on top of muscle relaxers, not only will you not have protective muscle spasms, but you will also not feel any pain related to the injury. By doing this, you will turn off all sensors for pain throughout your entire body.

Pain can actually work to your advantage if you understand it and can learn to work with it.

Within the body, there are thousands of things that happen every single second in order to coordinate all the daily actions of the body. Your brain receives three trillion pieces of information per second, to be exact. Information from every single cell in your body reports back up to the brain every single second. Your conscious or thinking brain can only interpret fifty pieces of information per second! That means the majority of information from your body never reaches your conscious brain![2]

So, how do we know what reaches your conscious brain and what does not? And what does the conscious brain pick to pay attention to?

Imagine what it must feel like to be the brain every second. It would be as though you are standing out in an open field and have 500 kids running up to you all at once, shouting to you about what they did that day or what they need. How do you decide which kids to listen to?

There are two different ways: The first way is that you are going to listen to the kids who run the fastest and get to you first. Then you are going to start scanning the crowd looking for emergencies.

2   James L. Chestnut, *The 14 Foundational Premises for the Scientific and Philosophical Validation of the Chiropractic Wellness Paradigm* (Victoria, BC: The Wellness Practice, 2003).

If you notice that a kid in the back of the group is bleeding from the head, you will listen to that kid over the one right next to you who is telling you about their pet cat.

Your brain does the same thing. Your brain interprets the first fifty bits of information it receives, as well as any urgent messages that come along.

This means that the pain you are feeling either:

1. Traveled faster than the other signals in your body to your brain, or
2. Is an urgent message that something is very wrong.

Because your conscious brain cannot interpret all of the signals coming from your body at once, it is possible that your severe lower back pain could be overshadowing another issue in your body. You can have pain or injuries that you do not feel because they are not as fast or as urgent as other injuries.

If pain becomes dull or numb, people often think that their injury is healed. This is not always true, as sometimes your brain will ignore a pain signal. The brain can get so tired of hearing the scream of pain that it cannot listen to it any longer.

If you have kids, I guarantee you have seen this happen: You are busy working on a project, and your kid goes, "Dad!" You know it's not urgent, so you ignore it. About a minute later, "Dad!" By the third time, there's a little more intensity in your kid's voice, "DAD!" The more you ignore the kid, the more they call for you. Pretty soon, it's: "Dad, Dad, Dad! Hey, DAD! Hello? Dad? Earth to Dad?" Except that screaming child calling for their dad is the pain signal.

Ever notice how some parents don't even hear their child anymore? They just continue grocery shopping as though the child is totally silent. I have witnessed this in the grocery store before, and I want to say to the parent, "Can you not hear your child?" But it turns out, the parent is really smart because, if this child continues to be ignored, eventually the child will get tired and stop trying to get their attention.

The same thing happens with pain. Your brain

has so many different signals to interpret that, after a while, it stops listening to them altogether. When your brain stops hearing the pain signals, you no longer feel pain. Your lower back can still be sending the pain signal, but the brain refuses to interpret it.

Since there are three trillion pieces of information per second that get sent to the brain, but only fifty pieces reach the conscious brain, how do we know what is happening inside our body? How do we know if things are working properly?

We can monitor what happens inside our bodies through blood pressure, blood work, breathing rate, samples of poop or urine, spinal x-rays, and chiropractic appointments.

Despite the brain's limited ability to read signals, people still have normal pain all of the time. People have normal headaches, normal low-back pain, normal sciatica. That means the headache that someone has 24/7 is one of those fifty signals that the brain can interpret every single second. What would your brain be able to interpret if it did not have to constantly interpret pain?

Remember, just because the pain is normal does not mean that you should have to live with pain for the rest of your life. The man at the beginning of this chapter who had normal headaches every day for twenty-five years was able to overcome his pain. Just because a certain type of pain is common in society does not mean that we *should* have it. Headaches are common, but that does not mean you should suffer from headaches.

When it becomes normal, that means we have accepted it as a part of our daily lives. We have given up on a solution. We have compromised. When we have daily headaches for twenty-five years, we begin to think that this is just how it's "supposed to be." We start to believe that our bodies are supposed to hurt and break down as we age. We believe that we just have bad genetics. Or it's just arthritis. Or that's just how we are. But that doesn't have to be true.

So many people live in constant pain that it has become normal and a common part of our culture.

REPAIR SHOP SUCCESS STORY: JOHN

In the winter of 2014, John came to my office shortly after I opened to address his severe neck pain. While going through his exam, I learned that he also had chronic lower back pain that limited many of his activities. His neck needed an adjustment like he suspected, but he also needed one in his lower back. When I moved to adjust his lower back first, he gave me a confused look and said in a very stern voice, "Don't you know that the issue is in my neck?"

I responded, "Yes, but we have to fix your lower back first in order to fix your neck."

He rolled his eyes and said, "You can do that, but only because I'm already here to get my neck fixed."

"Okay, lie down." I adjusted his lower back, then his neck. He rescheduled for the next week and left the office in a hurry.

Later that week, he came back in for his second visit. He walked in the door and gruffly asked, "What the hell did you do to me?" When I hear this from a patient, I'm never sure what made them say that.

I said, "Why do you ask?"

John then told me about how the lower back pain he had every day for eight years went away a few minutes after his adjustment and had not returned! At the time of my writing this, John still has not had any lower back pain since. This is amazing, and I am glad I was able to help John. But what if he had found an answer for his lower back pain when it first started? What if John had been adjusted when his lower back pain first appeared eight years ago? How would his life have been different if every day for eight years had been pain free? He should never have had to suffer from lower back pain for eight years.

WHY DO WE IGNORE THE "CHECK ENGINE" LIGHT?

Obviously, nobody wants to be in pain, so how and why does pain become normalized? I have found that normalized pain occurs when one or both of these two things has happened:

1. The person has pursued numerous different doctors and healers, changed their habits, and has still been unable to find relief from the pain. They eventually get tired of searching or run out of funds (or perhaps both) and give up. Instead of getting rid of their pain, they give up certain activities that exacerbate it. They might say, "If it hurts when I pick up my kids, then I just won't pick them up," and then it never hurts. They believe the injury is healed because the pain is controlled.

2. Their doctor told them that there is nothing that can be done to help them, and they will have to live with the pain—and the patient listened. The patient never got a second opinion. The patient agreed that this is "just how it has to be" or that "it must be my bad genes" or "I must be getting old."

If a doctor doesn't know *why* you have pain or can't help you get rid of your pain, then get a second opinion. You don't have to live with pain for the rest of your life just because one doctor said so. It simply means that they don't know how to help you with that specific condition. Remember, doctors are just people who are trying to help other people improve their lives. Anything a doctor tells you to do is merely their opinion. If a doctor doesn't know how to help you, I think they should tell you that they do not know and also help you find someone who can help you. (That's what I try to do for people anyway.)

Oftentimes, doctors are so specialized that they can't see the whole person and will miss the cause of the problem. High specialization in doctors can be helpful for certain conditions, but it can also be harmful because their scope of vision is so narrowed they no longer view their patient as a whole person with a whole body. A body that goes to work, volunteers at church, goes out with friends, is a child, parent, spouse, etc. Be sure to work with a doctor who views you as a whole individual, not a symptom.

Here is what is interesting to me: The majority of people I interact with who have daily pain do not expect it to ever get fixed. They just want some relief or a coping strategy so they can continue on with a normal life—in pain. People have settled for a life of constant headaches, constant lower back pain, constant knee pain, etc. They have given up on living pain free and cannot even imagine being healthy. Not because they do not *want* to be pain free but because everything they have tried, for months or perhaps even for years, has failed.

CHAPTER 2 ///

Why Did I Break Down?

There are two reasons for a car to break down: you either get in an accident, or you neglect routine maintenance on your car.

Whether you hit a deer or got rear-ended, an accident is called an accident for a reason. Besides, you not being there at that moment, there is nothing that could have been done to prevent it. It was just bad luck. But the good news is, once you fix the damage from the accident, your car will be up and running again.

We all have accidents where we hurt ourselves.

Accidents are unavoidable and will happen at some point. You could fall down the stairs, slip on a patch of ice, or injure yourself in any other way you can imagine. You were just in the wrong place at the wrong time. Once you get fixed, though, you are ready to go and do not have any other trouble.

Sometimes, it feels as though you had an accident, but then you find out that the reason your body broke down is that it was actually on the verge of a breakdown for weeks or maybe even months. You just didn't realize it because you were not performing the proper maintenance.

Using your car as an example: A belt could snap due to slow erosion that lasted weeks or maybe even months. There were no early warning signs or symptoms; the only way to detect this would have been to inspect that belt routinely and then notice that part of the belt looked dried out and cracked. There was no other way of knowing the belt was breaking down.

When the crack finally gets through the entire belt, then the belt snaps. Your car does not care if the belt snaps when you are at home, at the repair shop, or on the interstate. When the crack gets large enough, the belt will snap wherever your car happens to be. Hopefully, when the belt snaps, it does not damage anything else in the area.

If you had a good mechanic who was regularly checking over your car, they would have noticed that the belt was worn out and cracked. Your mechanic would have replaced the belt before it was ever an issue.

The same thing happens in people: something in them "snaps," and it is often blamed on a perceived accident, getting old, or bad genetics. For example, a person could bend forward to pick up a piece of paper and throw out their lower back. The act of picking up the paper did not do this, no matter how bad your lifting mechanics were at the time. This injury occurred because of neglect. The "belt," your injury, has been cracking for a long time, and it finally broke.

Whether you had an actual accident or suffered an injury due to neglect, the end result is pain, and now is the time to get it fixed up.

The best mechanic for the body is a chiropractor.

The main difference between healing from an accident and healing from neglect is the amount of time it will take in order to heal. The newer the injury, the quicker you will heal. The older the injury, the longer the healing process will take. It can be difficult to know how long that area has been injured. That belt could have started cracking one week ago, one month ago, one year ago, or twenty years ago. Even if you sought help immediately after the "belt" snapped, you might not have gotten help with the initial injury that took place. It was there for a long time without warning signs. Spinal X-rays are one way that chiropractors can tell you how long your spine has been injured.

"WON'T THE PAIN GO AWAY ON ITS OWN?"

Yes, anything can go away on its own. One way that humans are different from cars is that we have the ability to heal. When a car breaks down, you go and get it fixed because you know the car is incapable of healing on its own. When your body breaks down, you think, "Maybe it'll get better," and sometimes the pain does go away on its own. But how do you know if the pain went away because the body healed or because the brain stopped listening to the pain signals?

Whether your body truly healed or not has nothing to do with the severity of the injury. Every single ailment known to man has healed through spontaneous remission.[3] Spontaneous remission occurs when an injury or disease has healed completely on its own without any intervention—no medications, no surgeries, no acupuncture, no massages, nada. Some may have taken a few hours to heal; some may have taken years or decades. But there is at least one documented case of this for every single disease.

"WHY DOES THAT MATTER?"

Because it means you too can heal and live pain free if your body meets the right conditions. These are the questions you should be asking:

---

3 Brendan O'Regan, and Carlyle Hirschberg, *Spontaneous Remission: An Annotated Bibliography* (Petaluma, CA: Institute of Noetic Sciences, 1993).

- "What are the correct body conditions to allow healing?"
- "How do I get these conditions?"
- "How do I know if I'll be that case that heals on its own without any intervention?"
- "If I will be that case, how long will I have to wait for healing?"
- "Am I willing to have this pain for a day? A month? Twenty-five years?"
- "What if the pain doesn't go away?"
- "What if the pain causes other issues?"

I don't know about you, but I'm not that patient—and I don't want to gamble with my health. What if you don't try to intervene for an entire year, hoping the pain will heal on its own, but then it doesn't go away? Then you've lived a year of your life with unnecessary pain, and during that time the initial issue may have caused others to arise.

"WHEN SHOULD I GET A TUNE-UP?"

Generally, the sooner, the better, but getting to a chiropractor within the first thirty-six hours is key. Typically, the closer to your accident you can correct the injury, the faster you will heal. Remember, the injury date is when the "belt" *starts* to crack, not when the "belt" snaps.

When I begin to work with a patient in my office, it is similar to remodeling an old house. When you start a remodel, you often have one plan, but there are always a few bad surprises along the way (a water leak, cracked foundation, rotten floorboards, etc.).

This same thing often happens with an injury to the body. To have a properly functioning shoulder, for example, your pelvis has to be functioning properly as well because of the muscular connections between your shoulders and pelvis.

In my work, when a bad surprise arises, it always irritates me because it derails my original plan and delays the overall goal of pain-free living. I can no longer just address the initial complaint; I also have to go back and fix the original issue. If the first person had done this properly to begin with, then I would not have to spend as much time fixing it.

I often find people who tell me that they've had

this same injury for years or that, every January, they throw their lower back out on the first heavy snow. This is not how I want to see people. I don't want them to have to come and see me all the time for the same injury. If you are adjusted regularly and properly, it should fully fix the injury, so it does not keep recurring. Pain will only return through a new injury.

My goal is to fix the injuries well enough that people forget they were ever injured in the first place.

REPAIR SHOP SUCCESS STORY: EARL

When Earl came in for his first appointment, his X-rays were the worst I had ever seen, especially the ones of his neck. When a patient who has seen very few X-rays, says upon seeing one, "That doesn't look good," that's when you know it's bad. He was correct: It did not look good at all. His X-rays were full of arthritis, old injuries, and multiple segments I would not be able to adjust. Earl was a farmer, so his body had been put through a lot of abuse and neglect over the years. The worst time for him is planting and harvest season, where he and his teammates are working very long hours, spending a lot of time sitting forward in the tractor but looking backward. One thing that I have learned about farmers and many others in the Midwest is that they are not going to change their careers just because it is bad for their bodies.

Amazingly, Earl only needs a few adjustments each year now—before and after planting season, and before and after harvest season. Assuming he has no accidents, he will live pain free simply by adding four adjustments a year to his calendar.

Oftentimes, the hardest part is admitting the problem. The check engine light is on in your "car," and you can hear a loud clunking noise coming from the back every time you push on the brakes. Now is the time to decide: "What am I going to do about it?" Are you going to roll up the car windows, turn up the radio to drown out the sound of the problem, and hope maybe it'll go away? Maybe you'll get lucky and drive over a pothole, and it'll jostle that loose part back into place, right? Or maybe you could drive to a car shop and ask someone to check out the problem that day or, at the very least, make an appointment.

"WHAT IF I HAVE NO PAIN?"

"If I don't have any pain, does that mean I'm healthy and don't need to go to the doctor?"

Let me answer your question with another question: Have you ever known of someone who died of a heart attack? Yes, me too. I think that we all have. Have you ever been at that person's funeral when someone says, "I just don't understand why Joe had a heart attack. He was always healthy as a horse." I don't mean to sound like a total jerk, but last time I checked, people who are healthy as a horse don't just drop dead from a heart attack. One of the most common first signs of coronary heart disease is death by fatal heart attack,[4] meaning there is literally no known other warning sign before dying of these heart complications. To me, that's alarming.

---

4   CDC, "Heart Disease Facts," Centers for Disease Control, accessed
      October 23, 2020, https://www.cdc.gov/heartdisease/facts.htm.

Now, let's look at cancer for a minute: Did you ever hear of anyone who was suddenly diagnosed with stage-four cancer and told they only had a few months to live? It had already spread all over their body, and they didn't know anything about it until the recent diagnosis because they had no pain. If that same cancer case had caused symptoms that required medical assessment, then chances are it would have been found earlier. If you have to have cancer, it's best to find it early, so you can get treatment and make the needed lifestyle changes to heal. But what if you do not have pain indicating there is an underlying issue? How will you know you are sick or injured? This is why I find it important to go in for routine maintenance and, overall, to live a healthy lifestyle. The healthier you are, the better your body can function. The better your body functions, the lower your chances are of having a major health issue.

CHAPTER 3 ///

What Kind of Driver Are You?

The way you drive influences the future performance of your car. For the most part, there are two kinds of drivers: The first type is stop-and-go drivers. They accelerate as fast as possible at every green light only to throw on the brakes one block later at the next red light. The second type drives exactly the opposite way. Their driving is incredibly smooth, and it is even hard to tell if they are stepping on the brake or coasting to a slow stop.

Riding with the first type of driver gives me whiplash. I get a headache five minutes into the drive, and sometimes I even feel carsick. As you can imagine, the first driver's car needs more frequent maintenance, but it can always be repaired.

The same is true for the human body. The stop-and-go driver is the person who runs their body really hard until it gets overloaded and breaks down. These people are typically low on sleep, completely fueled by caffeine, and eat fast food in their car because they don't have time to sit down and eat. The only exercise they get is running back and forth to the car or around the grocery store. They are usually under a lot of stress at work and at home due to unrealistic demands and low-quality relationships.

Just like a car, the harder you run your body, the more maintenance it will need. You cannot usually change someone's driving habits. If they are the type of person to run their car or their body hard, then they will always be that way.

Typically, people know if they are running their bodies hard. They know they are a stop-and-go driver. That doesn't mean that habit has to change or that it will change. But they do need to do a better job of maintaining their body.

This person who runs their body hard eventually bends forward to pick up a piece of paper and their back goes out. Suddenly they are very injured, and they'll say, "But I didn't do anything!" or "It must be because I'm getting old." It's not that they didn't get injured, but rather that they were so distracted by everything else happening in their life that they did not realize they were slowly injuring themselves over time.

Every single thing that you encounter in your life, your spine and nervous system have to process. We all have good and bad stress continually piling up. Getting married. Having kids. Work. Working out. Poor posture. Good posture. Heavy lifting at work with and sometimes without good ergonomics. Eating healthy or unhealthy food. Negative and positive self-talk. The list goes on.

Everyone should work towards improving the health of their spine and nervous system. One way to do this is to go to the chiropractor "every 3,000 miles." For some, that might be twice a week. For others, it could be once a week, once a month, or once a quarter. It depends on how hard and how far you run your body.

If you drive ten hours every day on a road trip, you will rack up 3,000 miles really quickly. You will need more oil changes and maintenance driving like this, compared to only driving to the grocery store once a week. Not only do we have to consider *how* we drive our car but also how *far* we are driving.

"I NEVER GET MY OIL CHANGED"

Not needing a chiropractor is like having a car that never needs an oil change. Every single car needs regular oil changes. The difference is how often they get their oil changed and what kind of oil they put in the car, but that's it. The same with the chiropractor; the only difference is how often you will go and what you will need to work on. The better care you take of your body, the less work it will need by your chiropractor.

Here are some of the questions I ask myself to track how many miles (how much stress) I have run my body through recently:

- How much emotional stress have I had recently? (Emotional stress includes but is not limited to being overworked, depressed, anxious, fearful, angry, etc.)

- How much stress is work producing?
- How much stress are my family/friends producing?
- What has my diet been like this week?
- How many times have I exercised this week?
- Am I sleeping well? (This is a *very* important question because your body does the majority of healing when you sleep. If you are not sleeping well or for enough hours, be sure to get some more rest and you will automatically feel better.)
- Have any major events occurred in my life? (Examples include marriage, divorce, having kids, getting a promotion, getting fired, the death of a loved one, starting a new job, etc.)

If you can track these things on a weekly basis, it'll start to give you an idea of how soon you will hit your 3,000-mile marker. Know that your 3,000-mile mark might change at different times in your life and in different seasons.

Let's face it, though: no matter what kind of driver you are and how carefully you watch your mileage, you will still encounter a lot of stress. In 2020, we encountered more stress in one month than most people did during their entire lifetimes—even people like my grandparents who were born in the 1920s.

There are three avenues where stress can enter (or exit) our bodies:

1. Exercise
2. Fuel
3. Thoughts

EXERCISE

Your body is meant to get exercise. Your body actually craves exercise and physical labor. Now, when you have a lower back injury, I'm not expecting you to run a marathon or set records in the weight room, but you do still *need* exercise that is appropriate for that injury. The duration is dependent on you; you need to listen to your body to know when you should stop.

Years ago, medical doctors used to put patients on bed rest for injuries, but now this recommendation is very rare. The reason for this change is that they found bodies need motion to heal.[5]

Within the last year, I have had three patients who had broken their arms but walked around with no cast or sling on their arm. At first, I thought they just were not wearing the sling they were given. Then I was told that their medical doctors told them to move the arm as much as possible but not to use it to lift anything. The reasoning behind this is that it speeds healing time and the fracture heals two weeks faster than if it was in a sling or a cast.

The same is true for your spine. It is better to keep moving as much as possible. If it hurts to do something, quit moving. Also, avoid lifting heavy objects or lying in bed all day.

Movement acts as a pump, pushing swelling out of the injured area. It will also bring more healing to the area than if you had limited movement. Healing factors are the repair workers that get transported through the blood to the injured area

---

5   Donald Shelbourne, "Role of Early Motion in Healing Fractures and Ligaments Realized in the Last 25 Years," *Orthopedics Today* (2005).

in order to heal. With movement, the body actually sends more healing factors to the area in order to help you heal quicker.

Listen to your body, and let it tell you how much exercise it needs. Also, remember that while you are injured, the amount that it will need will change hour-to-hour and day-to-day. One hour you might only be able to walk around for two minutes, the next hour for six minutes, and maybe eighteen minutes after that. Trust me, your body will tell you if it needs more exercise; you'll start to feel antsy or restless. And if you've had too much exercise, it'll definitely tell you that as well, typically through more pain, spasms, or fatigue.

In addition to chiropractic care, here are three main exercises I recommend you do to help recover from and avoid lower back pain in the future:

1. **Walking:** Most people don't walk enough. You should walk for a minimum of one hour per day. Dividing your walking up through the day is more effective than taking one long walk. Be sure to practice walking forward and

backward. Walking backward helps the gluteus medius learn to fire. Engagement of the gluteus medius is key to releasing long-term lower back pain.[6]

2. **Planks:** A plank is when you hold the push-up position. If you can't hold the push-up position on the floor, go at an angle against a wall, a table, or even up the stairs. As you get stronger and advance, you can pick up your opposite arm and leg while keeping your back level. The plank is a full-body workout that will work your shoulders, chest, core, butt, and hamstrings.

3. **Primitive Squats:** As Americans age, we typically lose strength and flexibility in our legs and butt muscles. We squat every day when we sit down. Make it a goal to never use your hands to get up from a seated position. If that is easy for you, then you'll want to work on getting down into a deep or primitive squat. In a primitive squat, you are as deep in the squat as possible with your butt almost to the ground and feet flat on the floor. This squat is

---

6   N. A. Cooper, et al., "Prevalence of Gluteus Medius Weakness in People with Chronic Low Back Pain Compared to Healthy Controls," *European Spine Journal* 25, no. 4 (2016): 1258-1265.

instinctive in all of us when we are young. If you watch kids play, they will sit in a primal squat to play with a toy. Once the primitive squat is developed, then you want to work on staying in the squat longer, even walking around in the squat.

FUEL

Does the kind of fuel you put in your vehicle matter? If I put diesel into a car that does not take diesel, that is harmful to that car.

"What if I put food into my body that is harmful or unnecessary?"

When my grandparents had a farm, they didn't get their food anywhere else. They would butcher their own animals, grow and can their own organic vegetables, and drink raw milk from their own cows. They only went to the store for flour, sugar, or oats. This is an ideal way to live, but due to our modern lifestyles, very few of us can eat this way now.

About two years ago, I was told by a dairy farmer

that they are unable to eat any of the food from their farm because it's too dangerous. They can't drink the raw milk because of the large amounts of antibiotics given to the cows. They do not garden; they do not have chickens; crops (typically corn or beans) are too dangerous to eat until they are processed, so they are sold off. Most farms have turned into businesses that either grow crops or breed and fatten animals to a certain size. Then they're sold, and then they're turned into food. Some of the crops grown on our farms are not even used for food. Instead, they are turned into animal feed or ethanol.

Less and less of the food we eat comes directly from a farm. It goes from the farm through processing, and then we eat it.

My personal goal is to eat whole food from the earth or from animals. I do not follow any exact diet, but I do my best not to eat processed food. If my food does come in a package, I try not to eat anything with more than five ingredients. The better I fuel myself, the better off my body will be because the body literally breaks down food to power itself.

Your body is constantly building new cells to replace old or injured cells. The new cells are formed from the particles in the food you eat.

The old saying, "You are what you eat," is accurate. Would you rather your new cells be made from vegetables or from Twinkies? It takes your body seven to ten years to replace all its cells, so sticking to a healthy diet is key.

Eating well also gives your body the proper nutrients it needs to heal.

Two of the biggest issues in people's diets are sugar and gluten. Unfortunately, they can also be difficult for people to avoid when eating out or living on the go.

Cancer is fed by sugar.[7] If you have or have ever had cancer, you should never eat sugar again. If you are worried about getting cancer or feel as though you are predisposed in some way to getting cancer, then you should eliminate sugars

---

7   Chris Wark, *Chris Beat Cancer: A Comprehensive Plan for Healing Naturally* (New York City: Hay House, 2018).

from your diet. Not only is sugar good at feeding cancer, but sugar is also bad for the entire body.

To know if you are eating the proper foods, you will want to test your blood sugar before and after eating.

A simple way to do this is to buy a glucose monitor and test strips from a drugstore. A simple prick of the finger monitors how much sugar is in your food. The key is to test your blood sugar first thing in the morning to get a fasting blood sugar. Then also test your blood sugar one hour, two hours, and three hours after eating to assess how long it takes for your blood sugar to get back to the fasting level. You do not want your blood sugar to be spiked by the foods you are eating.[8] If your blood sugar does spike sky-high after eating, then you need to change what you eat.

Gluten has similar negative effects on health. Everyone has some sort of inflammatory response to it. But if you have never fully eliminated gluten

---

8 Alexis Shields, "Want to Know If Your Diet Is Healthy? Track Your Blood Sugar," Dr. Alexis Shields (2016), https://dralexisshields.com/blood-sugar.

from your diet, you probably do not recognize the inflammatory response in your body.

I can also confidently say that about 70 percent of people have a dairy intolerance.[9] It might not always end up in an upset stomach or diarrhea, but it can affect the body in other ways. Many of the kids I work with, who are ages six and up and still wet the bed at night, consume a high amount of dairy. When they cut down on dairy, the number of nights they wet the bed gets cut in half within a few days.

Nobody eats perfectly, but if we can improve how we eat, the body will have better resources to process. The food it breaks down then becomes a part of our cells. Every day, some cells die off, and new cells are born. This is how the body heals. If you can kill off all the unhealthy cells and grow new healthy cells, then your entire body make-up will change. The length of time this process takes varies. Some cells live for a few days, others for a month or more. The health of a new cell is depen-

---

9   David Neville, "Lactose Intolerance: Millions of Americans Don't Know They Have It," *Intermountain Healthcare*, https://intermountainhealthcare.org/blogs/topics/live-well/2017/07/lactose-intolerance/

dent upon what kind of food the body has broken down. It also depends on the nerve signaling from the brain about what kind of cell to make and what to make it out of.

What I have found helps me the most is only keeping good food in my house. When I buy junk from the grocery store, I eat junk. "Sift" is an app that I have found very helpful when in the grocery store. You scan the barcode on your food packaging, and the app tells you the ingredients and the health benefits or detriments of those particular ingredients.

The best foods to eat won't have a barcode to scan.

THOUGHTS

Did you ever fake sick as a kid in order to stay home from school? If you were like me, you definitely did. Here is what my experience was like.

I'd pretend that my nose was stuffed up, I had a cough, and I felt like I was going to throw up; then my parents would both leave for work. They would call me a few times throughout the day to see how I was doing, so I'd have to pick up the phone and sound sick. I would have to fake-cough and talk in a miserable voice over the phone, so they would continue to believe me. By their third call that day, I actually felt sick, and then I would *be* sick by the time they got home. I remember being upset about it because that morning I felt great! But the more I pretended to be sick, the sicker I would become. Then, the next day, I would actually stay home sick and typically have to go to the doctor.

This same thing happens each day with our thoughts! If you think positive, healing thoughts, your body will heal much faster and more efficiently. If you think negative thoughts while you are in pain, and you keep telling yourself that you will always be hurt and that it is something you just have to live with, it will be harder to get rid of the pain and heal from the injury.

Your thoughts manifest as realities in your body. You can choose to use those thoughts to get out of pain and improve your health, or you can use your thoughts to create more pain that will be detrimental to your health. I would hope that everyone reading this would want to utilize their thoughts to get out of pain and improve their health, but it is a lot harder than it sounds. It's easy to do this when you are not in pain. The more pain and worse health you are in, the harder it is to think positively and know that your thoughts are helping you in the long run.

The "white coat effect" is another common way that we can see how attitude affects the body. I'm sure you know someone who has experienced this, or you have experienced this yourself: the "white coat effect" occurs when somebody typically has normal blood pressure, but when they go to the doctor's office, their blood pressure always reads high due to their anxiety about being at the doctor's office.[10] Negative thoughts can impact the body outside the doctor's office, too. The trick is to understand that this happens and use it to our advantage to control or tweak our thoughts, so they do not affect our bodies negatively.

How our thoughts affect our healing has also

---

10 Briana Cobos, Kelly Haskard-Zolnierek, and Krista Howard, "White coat hypertension: improving the patient–health care practitioner relationship," *Psychology Research and Behavior Management* 8 (2015): 133–141.

been studied in cancer patients. Researchers have found that one of the main factors across all the different cancers—no matter if it's one that is easily curable or if it is a death sentence—that contributes to beating the cancer is a positive attitude.[11] Even folks who were given a horrible cancer diagnosis with only a few weeks to live are still alive five years later because they persevered with a positive mindset. They continued to live life and refused to plan their funeral or put their affairs in order. I figure if a positive attitude is important for cancer patients and if a negative attitude can make you sick when you aren't sick, then why not use your thoughts to help you heal? Why not envision yourself pain free and physically able to do what you want to do? Oftentimes, attitude is the missing link in the healing process.

We are all in control of our thoughts. The more positive your thoughts, the better off you will be. Here's one tip I've used in the past that I learned from my colleague, Dr. Lacey Book: On your smartphone, you are able to set multiple alarms per day. You can then change the name on the alarm. You could set an alarm to go off every hour

11 Wark, *Chris Beat Cancer*.

and tell you, "I am healthy" or "I am pain free." You can do this with any number of positive thoughts, so you can get multiple reminders throughout the day to help change your mindset.

REPAIR SHOP SUCCESS STORY: KEITH

Last summer, Keith came into my office for his first visit. Keith is a construction worker, and he said that his whole back hurts: his neck, middle back, and lower back. His appointment took place in the middle of the day, so he came into my office in his work clothes. I knew he must be in trouble because most construction workers are unable to leave work in the middle of the day, no matter how hurt they are. Keith came in and sat down, hunched forward. He said that he tried to work this morning, but he had such a high amount of pain throughout his entire back that he could not work. When looking at his back, I saw a twisting in his lower spine. I performed a standard adjustment at that location. When he got off the table, he stated that he already felt relieved and could tell this would help.

Two days later, Keith came back irritated and

upset with me. He snapped that he only had relief for about two hours after the adjustment. When I asked what happened that caused him to feel pain again, he said that he did not do any sort of movement, he did not lift anything, and he actually did not even go back to work. He simply went home. After some questioning, I found out that his dad had recently passed away. He said that every time he goes home, all he can think about is his dad's death. This is a case where the pain was not caused by a physical injury. It was caused by the mental and emotional stress of his dad's death. I continued to adjust him, but I also told him that his pain would not resolve until he grieved the death of his dad.

CHAPTER 4 //

How Often Does Your Car Break Down?

We all know that one person who always has car trouble. You know who I'm talking about. Their car always needs something fixed. This person gets their car fixed, and it seems to need another thing fixed a few weeks later. Their truck is all rusted out, cobbled together with different-colored side panels, and has a broken rear window covered in plastic and duct tape. Maybe this person is a friend of yours, a family member, or perhaps, it is you.

This person is forced to spend a lot of time and money on their car, and truth be told, they should probably be spending even more on it than they currently are. Not only is owning and fixing this car expensive, but it is also limiting.

Is this person able to get to work safely every day in this car? Could they drive across the country for a vacation? If they tried, how many times might they get stranded along the way?

The point is their car limits what they are able to do. Now, if they have the money, they can buy a new car. But if that broken-down, beat-up "car" is your *body*, you cannot go buy another one. Sure, you can get a knee replacement, but you can't replace the most important parts of your body: your brain, spinal cord, and spinal bones. This is why it is vital to take care of your spine. Without a healthy spine, your entire body will suffer.

It is important to know that there are limitations within your body. After having an injury for a period of time, your body can no longer repair itself. You are past the point of no return. It can partially improve, but if you are at this point, it will never go back to 100 percent mobility.

So, how do you know if it has been injured for too long? How do you know if you will never heal or if it will just take longer to heal? Nobody knows until you give the body a chance to work for you. I don't think any human ever really knows if that is the case for someone. I don't care who they are or what education they have; you never know what the body is capable of in terms of healing.

The hard part is being patient enough to give it the time and proper conditions to heal.

When I was a college student, I crashed my car head-on into a snowbank. I was too far in to get out. Luckily, a pick-up truck came by and pulled me out. I walked around the car, and unbelievably, there was no damage! So, I got in my car and kept driving as though nothing had happened. I didn't even tell my parents about it.

A week or two after the accident, I found myself in the driveway with my dad. He looked at my tires and wondered why the front tires weren't wearing evenly. I pled innocent. "Of course, I have no idea; I hardly know how a car runs, after all!" He finally told me that I must have run into something head-on and practically described the exact incident I had kept from him. He said, "If the tires were properly aligned, this would never have been an issue." I then had to pay for an alignment, which I should have done to start with, *and* new front tires!

This *exact* thing happens in the body: We have an accident, we emerge seemingly unscathed, and then we think the problem is fixed. Yes, the basic situation is fixed, but what underlying damage happened during the event?

I find this happens a lot with people with back pain and neck pain. They have no back pain at all, then all of a sudden, they are brushing their teeth at their bathroom sink when they get stuck in a forward-bending position. Or they have their head off to the side while brushing their hair, and their head and neck get caught that way. Obviously, brushing your teeth or hair doesn't cause you this stiffness, but your body had been out of alignment for so long, wearing improperly, that this stiffness became inevitable.

The wearing in your body is also the cause of arthritis. If you have a joint in the spine that wears properly, it will still wear out over time, but it will wear evenly. It will not change how the bone looks. Now, if one bone is twisted out of place and wears abnormally for *years*, then the body will start to reshape the bone to help it move better. It also reshapes the bone to eventually fuse the two vertebrae together that aren't moving properly. These are called bone spurs. While arthritis and bone spurs can cause trouble in the future, they are a very smart self-defense mechanism the body uses if the injury goes uncorrected for years. The best way to stop arthritis or slow down the process of it forming is to go to a chiropractor and have your bones realigned. That will help them wear properly and will also prevent them from fusing together.

You will also start to wear out your disc, the spacer between your bones, when your vertebrae are subluxated, or misaligned, over a long period of time. While it is true that you can have surgery to put in a fake disc, the motion unit is still not going to work correctly. The plastic surgical disc will wear out and create another problem. If you do end up needing a disc replacement, it is best to have the subluxation corrected before going through surgery, so then the vertebrae will move properly and protect the plastic surgical disc.

Every car needs a good mechanic. Chiropractors are mechanics for the spine.

If your spine does not function right, your body will not function right. A chiropractic clinic is the only place that helps correct an injury to the spine, so it doesn't keep flaring up over and over. Because, let's face it, who wants to continually break down? Most of us want to find a way to correct it over time. Nobody wants to be dependent on their chiropractor, medication, or physical therapy exercises.

CHAPTER 5 ///

Avoiding Breakdown

"I must be getting old."

This is something I hear from patients all of the time. The ironic thing about it is that I hear it from people who are ninety-two, twenty-two, and every age in between. Being old does not mean you have to be in pain or bad health.

Some of my healthiest patients are over eighty-five. They do not take medication, are active throughout the day, and perform chores around their home. Typically, the retired people I see are the busiest and healthiest people in my practice.

AN AGING EXAMPLE: HUBERT

Hubert was tall and lean. He had a full head of hair and very few wrinkles, and he wore small-framed glasses and flannel. I figured that he was no older than seventy-five. After viewing his date of birth on his intake form, I asked him if he wrote his birthdate down correctly because I did not believe that he was ninety-two. He looked like most of my seventy-year-old patients. He told me that he was, in fact, ninety-two but had worked hard to stay young.

He recently told me how sad he was because all of his friends were in nursing homes. He said that he couldn't believe he was the same age as them, not only because they look so old but also because they are unable to care for themselves or their house any longer. Hubert still lived at home and shoveled his own snow, unless the neighbor "boy," who was about forty-five, got to it first. He still drove a car and mowed his own lawn. He also walked five miles a day as long as there was no ice. I asked him how he stayed so active and healthy at his age, and he said the key was taking care of the body *right away* when it gets hurt.

It is because of people like Hubert that I do not let

anyone in my office blame their pain or stiffness on their age. In the United States, we are taught that our bodies are weak and that we are meant to be sick when, in fact, the opposite is true. Our bodies are actually designed to become stronger and healthier as we age.

REPAIR SHOP SUCCESS STORY: SHAWN

Fifty-two-year-old Shawn came into my office at the end of March. He owned a landscaping business and was in charge of mowing and trimming trees and bushes. Obviously, his busy time at work was during the spring and summer months. It was essential that he stayed able to work during this time. In February, he started having horrible pain in the middle of his back, down around the bottom part of his ribs, that made it hard to move. He said he tried everything to help with the pain. Shawn stated that he was in such bad pain that he wasn't sure if he'd be able to work at all that summer if it was unable to be fixed. Even riding in the car on the way to the jobs produced a large amount of pain from the jarring of being on the road.

I did my full history and exam on him. I took spine

X-rays and found one really bad spot right at the base of his rib cage. It was swollen and very tender to the touch. I adjusted him at that spot, and after his first visit, he reported that it was improved. He could ride in the car on the way to jobs pain free. He would still get some pain at the end of the day but said that he was 75 percent improved.

Within four visits, he felt 100 percent better and returned to work for the season. He has not had his back pain recur since. He now comes in about once every four weeks just to get it checked and make sure it's still okay. During one of his more recent visits, he exuded gratitude. Without my help, he said, he would have been forced to retire early, even though he could not afford to. Shawn told me he was now able to ride his bike again and use the older tractor at work. Previously, the older tractor was too rough to ride and would hurt his back. He also reported that his body could handle more work throughout the workday, and he had more energy overall.

There are lots of ways to treat the symptoms of pain. Many of these methods do just that: treat the symptoms *only*, allowing the pain to remain.

Sometimes treatment of the symptom is what we need for the moment, but it is important to make sure the underlying cause of the pain is also being addressed.

When people continue to reinjure themselves in the same area, this means, most of the time, it was never fully healed because they only treated the symptoms. If your only goal is to get out of pain, then the injury will never fully have time to heal.

When an injury doesn't have proper healing time, it's easy to do more damage and reinjure the area. Fully fixing the injury is difficult. You not only have to have the bone adjusted in the proper place but also ensure it is as strong as or even stronger than it was prior to the injury. Did you know that when you break a bone and it heals, it never rebreaks in exactly the same spot? That's because when the body healed that and laid down new bone, it actually added extra bone to make it stronger than before it broke. You need to do the same in your spine. This is done by stabilizing the area through chiropractic adjustments as well as living a healthy lifestyle.

I'm sure we all know someone who has a bad lower back. This person is always throwing out their back, but they never seem to hurt their neck. Sometimes they just throw their back out from sneezing, picking something up, a fall, or a car accident. However they injured their lower back, the same injury always results.

When someone injures themselves in the same spot over and over, I call this a "pain cycle." When you are injured, you are at the bottom or lowest point in the cycle. You start to move up the side of the cycle when you start to heal and feel better. At about the same time you're at the top of the cycle, you think you can coast. When you coast, you feel great, so you stop doing everything that helped you feel better. You stop doing all of the proper stuff to take care of the injury at home, and you stop coming to your chiropractic appointments. We all know that the only way to coast is to go downhill. Before you know it, you are back at the bottom of the cycle and in pain again. Now, you start going back in to get adjusted, and you start taking care of yourself at home, so you start to feel better. Then when you do, you stop again, so the cycle continues.

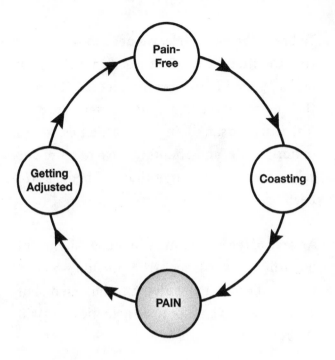

It might take a month for some people to get around this cycle. For others, they'll go through it every few months or even once a year.

When you injure your spine, it affects the disc, ligaments, tendons, muscles, nerves, etc. Your body also brings swelling and inflammation to the area to help it heal. Even after an adjustment, it can take up to six to eight weeks to fully heal the surrounding tissue to prevent reinjuring the same area.

To break the pain cycle, we need to remember that the first six to eight weeks are the most crucial period in the healing process. It is also the time when the injury feels better. When we feel better, we start doing more activities, return to normal life, and oftentimes, we reinjure ourselves because we forget that our body is still healing.

An area of the spine can be in proper alignment but still be a weak spot. Not only do we need to keep the alignment after an adjustment, but we also need to be sure to do activities that will strengthen the area as well.

Some strengthening activities for the lower back may include:

- Core strengthening activities like planks and reverse sit-ups
- Stretching, including proper warm-ups and cool-downs when working out
- Yoga and Pilates
- Foam rolling
- Using a tennis ball to work out muscle knots and break up adhesions

Ideally, we want the body strong enough to eliminate the weak points. Because just like water, stress will flow to the weakest area. Picture a river. A river is crooked because water always flows to the point of least resistance.

The same thing happens in the body. If you have a major injury in your spine, such as a compression fracture in one of your spinal bones, then that area of the spine will likely always be weaker. The compression fracture changes the shape of that individual spinal bone, and as a result, the shape of the entire spine has changed.

Most people do not get to the point of making their injury stronger than it was before the injury. There are many reasons that this happens, one of which is they do not come in for adjustments after the pain stops. I'm not saying that you have to come in for an adjustment once a week for the rest of your life. But if you get off the adjusting table and are pain free, then never come back, the chances are the original issue will not be fixed fully. After the pain ends, continual adjustments work to stabilize the injury. If you are only looking to get out of pain, then one adjustment to get you out of pain is all you need. If you want to stabilize and fully correct the injury, then a series of adjustments over time, paired with a healthy lifestyle, is key.

CARS MAKE WEIRD NOISES—DON'T IGNORE THEM

On the first beautiful day last spring, I decided to take my car out for a drive. I rolled down the windows and opened the sunroof. As I started to drive, I could hear my car making horrible noises that I knew were not normal. So, what did I do? Obviously, I rolled up the windows and turned up the music!

I hope you don't believe that because that's definitely not what I did! I recorded the noise and took the car into the repair shop the next day to get fixed.

When our body starts clunking and causing us pain, it's too easy to ignore the issue. There are a lot of things out there that can help us ignore pain in the body.

Some of them are:

- Over-the-counter painkillers
- Muscle relaxers and prescription painkillers
- Old prescription medication from previous injuries, surgeries, or health issues
- Alcohol
- Illegal drugs
- Massages
- Electric stimulation, using four adhesive pads around the painful muscles
- Inversion tables
- *Biofreeze*
- *IcyHot*

All of these things can relieve pain, but so can an adjustment. So why not just buy a cheap bottle of ibuprofen and pop a bunch of those instead of getting adjusted? Or why not get drunk? High on drugs? Slather on *IcyHot*? Have your kid walk on your back? Most of the time, these strategies are cheaper than an adjustment. But a series of adjustments will correct the problem in the long term and help people avoid continual injury.

Oftentimes, finding ways to eliminate the pain will cause not only more damage down the road but also a separate problem. For example, if you take a lot of painkillers, you may damage your kidneys in thirty years; then you will be in numbed pain *and* have a kidney problem to take care of. Why trade one issue in for another?

Being out of pain is great, and these strategies have their place in the healing process, but you will eventually become dependent on these things if you live in a constant state of pain. With adjustments to your spine, you are able to help the pain as well as correct the injury, so it does not keep recurring.

Let's fix the big issues while they're small issues. We want to fix the issues, not roll up the windows and turn on the radio.

How far and how hard you run your body is the part I have no control over as your chiropractor. You are in total control of how hard you run your body and how much negative stress you let build up. The key is that when you hit the 3,000-mile mark, you schedule a tune-up, so we can get you right back on the road. The most difficult part about this is that your body does not come with an odometer to track the miles like a vehicle does. So, we have to find other ways to track the miles.

All of the bad stress is constantly building up and working towards lowering your stress threshold, leaving you more susceptible to getting sick and injured. The good news is you do not have to wait until your stress level gets to capacity to lower it. For example, if you have a swimming pool that is plugged and a water hose is filling the pool, then eventually the pool will run over. To keep this from happening, you either need to pull the plug in the pool or shut off the water. It's the same with stress in your life. You can either lower the amount of stress in your life or find ways to get rid of your stress. For most people, it is easier to find ways to deal with your current stress than it is to lower the amount of bad stress you encounter daily.

We all get caught up in our own lifestyle, and it's often difficult to step away from that lifestyle and identify what needs to be changed. When we know what needs to be changed, oftentimes we will not change it because it's just too difficult. It is much easier to maintain your fast-paced life than deal with the stress it brings.

One way to eliminate stress is to get adjusted by

your chiropractor. Other great ways to reduce stress are to:

- Work out using a combination of cardio and strength (this is the best)
- Meditate or say daily affirmations
- Do yoga
- Do body work like massages, acupuncture, reiki, etc.
- Eat more veggies, meat, and fruit, and fewer carbs and desserts
- Increase your water intake

My goal with patients is not to take away anything you do in your daily life or make you compromise your happiness. I want to help you reduce your stress, and perhaps more importantly, I want to increase the amount of stress that your body can handle. The healthier your spine is, the more stress your body can handle.

For the body to fully heal, it needs to cultivate the right environment. When creating the correct healing environment inside of your body, the first necessity is proper nervous system function. If the brain is able to send proper signals out to the body to tell it what to do, the body will be able to function perfectly. This is why it is vital to regularly go to a chiropractor. Regular adjustments to the spine will make sure the nervous system is working properly.

When the nervous system works well, you may still have pain, but the body will be able to recover from it on its own. It couldn't recover before because the spine wasn't functioning right to start with. This is why I always start repairing my health at the chiropractor and move on from there. I figure that if the adjustment cannot realign my spine, then we have a huge issue because that means my body is not working properly. I need a whole different sort of intervention. The important thing when going to the chiropractor is not to just go until your spine is fully stabilized. Sometimes I adjust someone who has been in horrible pain for a month. Immediately after the adjustment, the pain is gone. That is great, but the trick is that vertebra was sitting out of place for at least a month, maybe two months, or possibly even years. So, the damage to the disc, ligaments, tendons, and muscles is not fully corrected. They will heal on their own, but since they are still injured, they might cause that subluxated bone to pull back out of place before it fully heals.

Think about it like this: Say you have a tomato plant, and at the beginning of the growing season, you can see your plant is budding ten small tomatoes. If you pluck off half of the tomatoes early in the season, the remaining five tomatoes will end up being bigger and tastier than if you had left all ten on the plant. Picking some tomatoes creates more room for the remaining tomatoes to grow. No matter how many tomatoes on the plant, it will always put 100 percent of its power into growing tomatoes. You will get bigger and better tomatoes if it grows five versus ten tomatoes.

This same principle is true for the body. The body has 100 percent healing energy within. If the body has ten different injuries or diseases to heal, then its healing power gets divided into ten different places, so each place only receives 10 percent healing power. If the body has five injuries or diseases to heal, then each gets 20 percent; if it has two to heal, then each gets 50 percent of the healing power.

This is why the healthier you are and the fewer injuries that you have, the faster your body will heal.

My goal is to get you to a healthy starting place, so when you do catch that cold or you fall down a flight of stairs, you will recover quickly and be back to 100 percent in no time.

Your body wants to function normally and be in a state of health. One of the best things about chiropractic care is that it allows the body to heal exactly how it needs to heal. Once the spine is well adjusted and in alignment, it will begin to heal.

The body never does anything by accident. It doesn't create pain or go out of alignment for no reason. When we get the spine and nervous system working properly, your body will work correctly. When your body is working correctly, you will not only notice that your pain is gone, but you'll also notice other benefits like increased immune function, better sleep, better ability to focus, better balance, and more. The benefits of a body functioning at 100 percent are endless.

"CAN I JUST ADJUST MYSELF?"

The short answer is no. Oftentimes, people think that they are adjusting themselves because they can move in a certain way to make their spine pop. But that's not an adjustment. That simply means that area of your spine has more mobility than other areas.

When you pop your own spine, you get lots of different pops. For every pop, a rush of endorphins gets released. Endorphins make you happy. If you pop one bone, you get one "shot" of endorphins. If you pop two bones, you'll get two. And so on.

Popping your own spine typically does not target the bone that needs the adjustment. Let me explain: most likely, the reason you feel like you need an adjustment is that you are in pain, feel tight, or have some limited mobility.

The spinal bone that needs adjusting has been out of alignment and stuck longer than you have felt those symptoms. This misaligned spinal bone ("subluxation" is the technical word) is surrounded by inflammation, swelling, and muscle spasms. The misaligned or subluxated spinal bone does not move easily, not even for the chiropractor.

When you twist your neck or lower back or have someone else lift you up or walk on your back, the target bone won't move because the inflammation, swelling, and muscle spasms keep it in its misaligned state to avoid any further damage. What you hear when you pop your neck is the healthy, well-aligned spinal bones surrounding the misalignment crack. At some point, this will cause damage to the healthy spinal bones.

Popping your own spine too often can cause damage. If you are currently popping your own spine, do your best to stop. It will be difficult to stop because:

1. Your back will feel really tight when you stop popping it multiple times per day. (That is okay and a normal thing to have happen.)
2. You will no longer get a blast of endorphins every time you pop your back.

Here's the thing, though: Those endorphins will spike you up and make you feel great, but then you will crash, similarly to when you are on a sugar high. As soon as you crash, you have to search for more sugar. Most people are actually addicted to the endorphin high, so you will have to slowly break the addiction. Most people cannot quit cold turkey. Actually, most people who pop their spine on a regular basis do not even realize how often they do it because it's a habit or a nervous tic they have.

When I see someone in my office who pops their spine all of the time, they typically get confused at the end of the visit because the parts of the spine I work on are either above or below the parts of the spine that they pop. This is because they are popping the compensation, or the healthy spinal bone, and not the subluxation or injured area. If you allow your chiropractor to pop your back in the right way and actually reposition the bone (instead of just stimulating the area), then you will experience true healing.

When patients come to my office to get adjusted, I always adjust them from behind. I push forward on their backs. I'm never pushing from the side or the front of their bodies. Unless they have freakishly long arms that allow them to reach all the way around their back and achieve the proper angle, there is no way they could adjust themselves.

Even if your arms could reach that far, it's impossible to check yourself to figure out if and where you even need an adjustment. Even when I need an adjustment—even when I'm almost positive that I understand the issue based on my symptoms and what I can feel in my own spine—I am almost always wrong when I go in to see my chiropractor. We just cannot do it ourselves.

Now, if you are doing something within your normal routine—let's say you roll over in bed, and your back pops—that's fine. That is going to happen. What I don't want you doing is putting any pressure onto your spine to pop it, contorting your spine so it will pop, or having someone walk on your back or lift you up to pop your spine. The more you do these things, the more you'll need a chiropractor. It might not be immediately, but eventually it will do damage to your spine.

CHAPTER 6 //

Increasing Your Tire(d) Pressure

I do not want to ever adjust you again.

This does not mean we wrap you in bubble wrap to keep you from ever needing another adjustment. Instead, we are going to increase your body's ability to handle and process stress. The body's ability to handle and process stress is called adaptation. The better your body can adapt to the world around you, the fewer adjustments you will need.

Nobody wants to be dependent upon medication, surgery, or weekly chiropractor appointments. My goal is to build up the tolerance or threshold in your body, so you are able to handle more stress.

The way to build up your threshold is to have a properly functioning spine. The better your spine functions, the higher your stress threshold.

This means that you have two jobs for the rest of your life. The first one is to find ways to reduce the stress you put on your body. You will never eliminate all of the stress in your life, but it can be reduced.

Your second job is to *keep* your spine healthy so your body can process higher amounts of stress. The main way to improve the health of your spine is through chiropractic adjustments.

Again, the goal is to never need another adjustment.

It is impossible to lift and move properly all the time. Your body *can* handle the stress of improper lifting, eating toxic food, and thinking negative thoughts—just not all the time.

Yes, I want you to lift or move your body effectively

and appropriately with proper ergonomics when you can. But you cannot lift something perfectly all of the time. When you cannot lift properly, I want your body to be able to handle that stress.

REPAIR SHOP SUCCESS STORY: BRANDON

My patient Brandon is a great example of this. Brandon is a fifty-five-year-old car mechanic in town. He kept hurting his lower back, middle back, and sometimes his neck due to his work. His injuries typically happened when he had to crawl into an awkward position in a car to fix it. (If you don't work on cars for a living, watch the mechanic next time. They are bending over while also twisting, pulling on a stuck part, etc. In a way, they are contortionists.)

Brandon got to the point where his last chiropractor started to limit every movement that caused an injury. If he hurt his lower back by picking up a tire by himself, he was no longer allowed to do that. The other chiropractor in town eventually told him his job was too hard on his body, that he should consider another career or retire. He was unable to retire and didn't know how to do anything other than work on cars. To him, neither of those were an option.

When Brandon came to my office for his first adjustment, he said that he *has* to be able to fully perform his job, move in all directions, not have restrictions, *and* live pain free.

I adjusted him and stabilized his spine. Now that his spine functions properly, Brandon is able to work without worrying about what position his body is in. He can simply focus on his work.

Does he still get hurt? Sometimes. Accidents will happen; that's why they are called accidents. But when he does get hurt, he is able to heal quickly and go back to work the same day.

The key to becoming pain free like Brandon is getting the spine functioning normally under chiropractic care, so it can better adapt to the stress you put it under.

Remember, your body is a self-regulating and self-healing organism. Your body *wants* to be healthy. Your body always works properly.

Even pain, sickness, and disease are all proper functions.

The choice is yours. You can only go to the chiropractor when you are hurt, or you can go in regularly for prevention. Would you rather take your car in for oil changes every three thousand miles or let it run out of oil and do long-term damage to the car?

Hopefully, you won't ever need a chiropractor to adjust you again. But if you think or feel like your spine is injured, not functioning properly, or that something is off, then go and get it checked by a chiropractor right away. If it needs work, then a quick adjustment can be made to get you back in the game. If it doesn't need work, then at least we know the spine is healthy and that it will heal on its own. For Americans living the standard American life, their bodies can usually only handle the build-up of stress for one month before they need an adjustment.

Currently, the record time at my office for not needing an adjustment is two years. Think you can break it?

Conclusion

Anyone can have a small slip or fall that injures their body temporarily, making them unable to work without taking something to dull the pain and unable to do any of their hobbies without pain.

Imagine a world where people recovered from injures quickly. Imagine a place where nobody ever thought about taking daily pain medications, where the majority of people were healthy and sickness was rare. Imagine the things that society could accomplish then.

Think of what our towns would be like if people did not have to decide what they wanted to do based on the limitations of their health and their pain. If they wanted to do something, then they would just do it because their body could handle the stress.

This is the world I dream about. This is the world I am working towards.

Everyone I see in my office has a limitation in their body, an injury, or disease in their body that is limiting their quality of life. But what if we could eliminate all of them? I am not saying that you will never have a car accident or never fall down the stairs. You will. But it is my hope for you that when that happens, you can come to my office, get adjusted, quickly heal, and forget that it ever happened, making it a speed bump instead of a detour that takes years.

I cannot do this alone. I need the help of others to help spread my vision. The world I am dreaming of is so far from what people can imagine and what the normal American experiences, so I need your help spreading the word. I know that you want to feel better and be healthier. You also probably even want that cranky co-worker of yours to start to feel better too, even if it's merely so you don't have to put up with their complaining anymore. Let's stop the negativity by helping people feel better. If we feel better, then we can all be better humans.

My challenge to you is to find one other person who needs to read this book. Find one person this book could help. I want you to give them your copy of the book or get a free copy from me to give to them. Have them read it.

If you think that chiropractic care could help either you, your family, friends, or co-workers, please call me for a free consultation at my office. This will allow me to review the case and see if I can help get you or your loved ones (or frenemies) out of pain. If I cannot help them, then I will find somebody who can.

Acknowledgments

I would like to thank my family and friends who have always supported and encouraged me through my work—especially my parents, Linda and Charlie, and my brother, Adam.

I would also like to thank all the chiropractors who came before me and taught me this work. Without them, none of this would be possible. I would like to especially thank Dr. Alex Cox for his continued support and encouragement over the years.

A big thank you to all the patients I get to work with at my office on a daily basis. It truly is an honor to work with all of you. You inspire me to be a better person.

And, of course, thanks to the Scribe team for helping me make this book a reality.

About the Author

DR. LAURIE MEINHOLZ was raised in Madison, Wisconsin. She is a 2008 graduate of Luther College, where she studied theater/dance and psychology. It was during her time at Luther College and through her study in dance that she knew she wanted to pursue a career centered in the body. A few years after graduation from Luther, Dr. Laurie decided to become a chiropractor. While at Palmer College, she was president of the largest club on campus, the Gonstead Club. She graduated from Palmer College of Chiropractic in 2013 and was one of four students in her class nominated for the Virgil Strang Philosophy Award. Dr. Laurie has over 500 extra hours of study in Gonstead Chiropractic.

She has always loved Decorah, as it has always felt like home. After graduation from Palmer in 2013, she opened her office, Nordic Chiropractic, in Downtown Decorah.

Dr. Laurie currently serves on the board of the International Federation of Chiropractors and Organizations (IFCO). She is also a visionary regent of Sherman College of Chiropractic, as well as a regent of the Australian Spinal Research Foundation. Dr. Laurie loves to mentor current chiropractic students and new graduates, helping them learn the art of adjustment.

It is important to Dr. Laurie to find multiple ways to give back to the community. Dr. Laurie donates 100 percent of the profits from Nordic Chiropractic to local charities that are nominated by her patients. Dr. Laurie served on the Nordic Fest board for four years and was the president of the board in 2017. She also started the Decorah Running Club in 2019 to help runners connect and support each other.

CPSIA information can be obtained
at www.ICGtesting.com
Printed in the USA
FSHW011459030321
79116FS